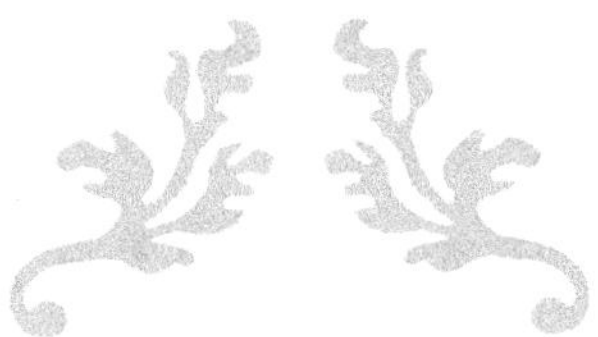

The Healing Power of Nature:

How Spending Time Outdoors Can Improve Mental Health

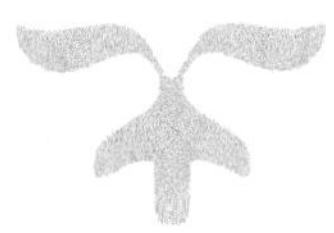

Preface:

As we go through our daily lives, we are bombarded with stress, distractions, and pressures that can take a toll on our mental health. But what if we told you that there is a simple solution that can improve our well-being and bring us a sense of peace and calm? This solution is nature.

Nature has been an essential part of human existence for centuries. It has been a source of inspiration, beauty, and sustenance. However, in recent years, our lives have become more hectic and disconnected from the natural world. This disconnection has contributed to a rise in mental health issues such as anxiety, depression, and stress-related disorders.

This book explores the healing power of nature and how spending time in nature can benefit our mental health. The book provides a comprehensive overview of the scientific research that supports the benefits of nature, as well as practical tips and strategies for incorporating nature into our daily lives.

The chapters in this book cover a range of topics, from the science behind nature to the benefits of nature for specific mental health conditions. We also explore the healing power of gardening, the importance of social connection in nature, and how to make nature a part of our daily routine.

Our hope is that this book will inspire readers to reconnect with nature and improve their mental health and well-being. We believe that by prioritizing our relationship with nature, we can find a sense of peace, joy, and balance in our lives.

We would like to thank our contributors for their expertise and insights, as well as our readers for joining us on this journey to explore the healing power of nature.

About the Author:

Dr. Sarah Kim is a mental health professional with a passion for exploring the therapeutic benefits of nature. She holds a Doctorate in Psychology and has over 10 years of experience working in various mental health settings.

Dr. Kim has always been drawn to nature, and over the years, she has witnessed the powerful impact that spending time outdoors can have on mental health. She has conducted extensive research on the topic and has worked with patients to incorporate nature into their therapy sessions.

In addition to her clinical work, Dr. Kim is also an advocate for environmental conservation and the protection of natural spaces. She believes that our connection to nature is essential for our mental and physical well-being, and that by prioritizing this connection, we can create a more sustainable and fulfilling future.

Through her writing and speaking engagements, Dr. Kim hopes to inspire others to prioritize their relationship with nature and to reap the benefits of spending time outdoors. She currently resides in the Pacific Northwest with her family and enjoys hiking, gardening, and exploring the natural beauty of the region.

Table of Contents

Introduction:

Nature has been an essential part of human existence since the dawn of time. It has provided us with food, shelter, and resources for survival. However, as we have become more urbanized and technologically advanced, our connection to nature has weakened. Today, many people spend the majority of their time indoors, disconnected from the natural world. This disconnection has come at a cost to our mental health, with rates of anxiety, depression, and other mental health conditions on the rise.

In recent years, there has been a growing interest in the healing power of nature. Research has shown that spending time in nature can have significant benefits for mental health, including reducing stress, improving mood, and promoting overall well-being. Nature-based therapy, such as ecotherapy and horticultural therapy, is becoming increasingly popular as a treatment option for mental health conditions.

The Healing Power of Nature: How Spending Time Outdoors Can Improve Mental Health is a book that explores the connection between nature and mental health. In this book, we will delve into the science behind the healing power of nature, examining how spending time in nature affects the brain and promotes mental wellness. We will explore the benefits of outdoor activities for specific mental health conditions, including anxiety, depression, ADHD, and ADD. We will also provide practical tips for incorporating nature into daily life, making it accessible to everyone.

The purpose of this book is to raise awareness of the benefits of nature for mental health and to provide readers with the knowledge and tools to incorporate nature into their own lives. By the end of this book, readers will have a better understanding of the science behind nature therapy, the benefits of nature for specific mental health conditions, and practical strategies for incorporating nature into daily life.

Whether you are struggling with a mental health condition or simply looking to improve your overall well-being, this book will provide you with the knowledge and inspiration to harness the healing power of nature. Let's take a step outside and reconnect with the natural world for improved mental health and wellness.

Chapter 1: The Science Behind Nature

Humans have an innate connection to the natural world. We have lived in close proximity to nature for thousands of years, and our well-being has been closely tied to the natural environment. However, in today's modern world, we spend less time in nature than ever before, and this disconnect has come at a cost to our mental health. In recent years, there has been a growing interest in the science behind nature therapy and its potential benefits for mental health.

Biophilia: Our Innate Connection to Nature

The concept of biophilia, coined by biologist E.O. Wilson, refers to the innate tendency for humans to seek connections with nature. Biophilia is deeply ingrained in our biology, and it has been shown that exposure to nature can promote physical and mental health.

Research has shown that even brief exposure to nature can improve mood, reduce stress, and improve cognitive function.

The Impact of Nature on the Brain

Spending time in nature has been shown to have a significant impact on the brain. Studies have shown that exposure to nature can reduce cortisol levels, the hormone associated with stress, and increase the production of endorphins, the body's natural "feel-good" chemicals. Exposure to nature has also been shown to improve cognitive function, memory, and attention.

Nature-Based Therapies

Nature-based therapies, such as ecotherapy and horticultural therapy, are becoming increasingly popular as treatment options for mental health conditions. These therapies involve spending time in nature and engaging in activities such as gardening, hiking, and animal-assisted therapy. Research has shown that these therapies can be effective treatments for conditions such as anxiety, depression, ADHD, and ADD.

The Importance of Green Spaces

The concept of environmental psychology examines the relationship between people and their physical environment. This field of study has shown that our surroundings can have a significant impact on our mental health and well-being. Urbanization and the decline of green spaces have led to an increase in mental health conditions such as anxiety and depression. However, the creation of green spaces in urban areas can have a significant positive impact on mental health.

Conclusion

In conclusion, this chapter has explored the science behind nature therapy and the potential benefits of spending time in nature for mental health. We have discussed the concept of biophilia and how exposure to nature can promote physical and mental health. We have examined the impact of nature on the brain, including its ability to reduce stress, improve mood, and promote cognitive function. We have also discussed the benefits of nature-based therapies and the importance of green spaces for mental health. This knowledge will lay the foundation for the practical tips and strategies provided in later chapters for incorporating nature into daily life for improved mental health and well-being.

Chapter 2: The Benefits of Nature for Anxiety and Depression

Anxiety and depression are two of the most common mental health conditions, affecting millions of people worldwide. While traditional treatments such as medication and therapy can be effective, many people are turning to nature-based therapies as a way to alleviate symptoms and improve their overall well-being.

Reduced Symptoms of Anxiety

Studies have shown that spending time in nature can reduce symptoms of anxiety. One study found that a group of individuals with anxiety who spent time in a forest had lower levels of anxiety and improved mood compared to a control group who spent time in an urban environment. Another study found that spending time in nature can improve heart rate variability, which is a measure of the body's ability to respond to stress.

Improved Mood and Reduced Symptoms of Depression

Depression is another mental health condition that can be alleviated by spending time in nature. A study published in the Journal of Affective Disorders found that people who spent time in nature had significantly lower levels of depression compared to those who spent time in an urban environment. Another study found that spending time in a green environment, such as a park or forest, can improve mood and reduce symptoms of depression.

Boosted Self-Esteem and Sense of Well-Being

Spending time in nature can also improve self-esteem and a sense of well-being. A study published in the Journal of Environmental Psychology found that people who spent time in nature had higher self-esteem and were more likely to feel connected to their surroundings. Another study found that people who walked in a natural setting had higher levels of well-being compared to those who walked in an urban environment.

Increased Social Interaction

Spending time in nature can also increase social interaction, which is important for people with mental health conditions such as anxiety and depression. Studies have shown that people who spend time in nature are more likely to engage in social interactions and feel a greater sense of connection to others.

Conclusion

In conclusion, this chapter has explored the benefits of spending time in nature for anxiety and depression. We have discussed how exposure to nature can reduce symptoms of anxiety and depression, improve mood and self-esteem, and increase social interaction. These findings provide strong evidence for the use of nature-based therapies as an effective treatment for mental health conditions. By incorporating nature into daily life, individuals can experience these benefits and improve their overall well-being. The next chapter will provide practical tips and strategies for incorporating nature into daily life for improved mental health.

Chapter 3: Nature and Stress Reduction

Stress is a common and often unavoidable part of life, and it can have negative effects on both physical and mental health. However, research has shown that spending time in nature can be an effective way to reduce stress levels and improve overall well-being. This chapter will explore the relationship between nature and stress reduction, as well as practical tips for incorporating nature into daily life to manage stress.

The Science Behind Stress and Nature

Stress is the body's response to a perceived threat, and it can lead to a variety of physical and mental health problems if left unmanaged. Studies have shown that spending time in nature can reduce levels of cortisol, the hormone associated with stress, and promote feelings of relaxation and calmness.

One study published in the International Journal of Environmental Research and Public Health found that spending time in a natural environment can reduce the physiological markers of stress, such as heart rate and blood pressure. Another study found that individuals who spent time in nature had a lower level of perceived stress compared to those who spent time in an urban environment.

The Benefits of Nature for Stress Reduction

Nature provides a range of benefits for stress reduction, including:

1. Improved mood: Spending time in nature can promote feelings of happiness and well-being, which can help counteract the negative effects of stress.
2. Increased physical activity: Many outdoor activities, such as hiking or gardening, can provide a source of physical exercise, which can reduce stress levels and improve overall health.
3. Sensory stimulation: The sights, sounds, and smells of nature can provide a calming and relaxing environment, reducing stress levels.
4. Social interaction: Spending time in nature can provide opportunities for social interaction and connection with others, which can be beneficial for reducing stress and improving mental health.

Incorporating Nature into Daily Life

There are many practical ways to incorporate nature into daily life for stress reduction, such as:

1. Spending time in local parks or green spaces
2. Gardening or spending time in a backyard or balcony garden
3. Taking a walk in a natural environment
4. Practicing outdoor yoga or meditation
5. Engaging in outdoor hobbies, such as birdwatching or photography

Conclusion

In conclusion, this chapter has explored the relationship between nature and stress reduction. We have discussed the scientific evidence supporting the use of nature as a way to reduce stress levels and improve overall well-being. We have also provided practical tips for incorporating nature into daily life to manage stress. By making nature a regular part of daily life, individuals can experience the many benefits of nature and improve their mental and physical health. The next chapter will explore the relationship between nature and sleep, and how spending time in nature can improve sleep quality.

Chapter 4: The Impact of Nature on ADHD and ADD

Attention Deficit Hyperactivity Disorder (ADHD) and Attention Deficit Disorder (ADD) are common neurodevelopmental disorders that can cause difficulties with attention, impulse control, and hyperactivity. While medication and therapy are commonly used to manage symptoms, research has shown that spending time in nature can also have a positive impact on individuals with ADHD and ADD. This chapter will explore the relationship between nature and ADHD/ADD, and how spending time in nature can improve symptoms.

The Science Behind Nature and ADHD/ADD

Studies have shown that spending time in nature can improve symptoms of ADHD and ADD. One study published in the Journal of Attention Disorders found that children with ADHD who spent time in natural environments had reduced symptoms of inattention and hyperactivity compared to those who spent time in built environments. Another study found that children with ADHD who engaged in outdoor activities experienced improvements in cognitive function and attention.

The Benefits of Nature for ADHD/ADD

Nature provides a range of benefits for individuals with ADHD and ADD, including:

1. Reduced symptoms: Spending time in nature can help reduce symptoms of inattention, impulsivity, and hyperactivity.
2. Improved cognitive function: Nature provides a stimulating environment that can improve cognitive function, including attention and memory.
3. Increased physical activity: Many outdoor activities, such as hiking or biking, can provide a source of physical exercise, which can reduce symptoms and improve overall health.
4. Sensory stimulation: The sights, sounds, and smells of nature can provide a calming and relaxing environment, which can reduce symptoms of ADHD and ADD.

Incorporating Nature into ADHD/ADD Treatment

Nature can be incorporated into ADHD/ADD treatment in a variety of ways, including:

1. Outdoor therapy: Therapeutic sessions held in natural environments can help individuals with ADHD/ADD manage symptoms and improve overall well-being.
2. Nature-based interventions: Nature-based interventions, such as wilderness therapy or adventure therapy, can help individuals with ADHD/ADD build skills and reduce symptoms.
3. Spending time in nature: Simply spending time in natural environments, such as local parks or hiking trails, can provide a range of benefits for individuals with ADHD/ADD.

Conclusion

In conclusion, this chapter has explored the relationship between nature and ADHD/ADD. We have discussed the scientific evidence supporting the use of nature as a way to reduce symptoms of ADHD and ADD. We have also provided practical ways to incorporate nature into ADHD/ADD treatment, such as outdoor therapy and spending time in nature. By including nature in ADHD/ADD treatment plans, individuals can experience the many benefits of nature and improve their overall well-being. The next chapter will explore the relationship between nature and creativity, and how spending time in nature can improve creative thinking.

Chapter 5: The Healing Power of Gardening

Gardening has been a popular pastime for centuries, but it also has significant mental health benefits. In this chapter, we will explore the therapeutic benefits of gardening and how it can help improve mental health.

The Therapeutic Benefits of Gardening

Gardening has a range of therapeutic benefits, including:

1. Stress reduction: Gardening has been shown to reduce stress and promote relaxation. It provides a calming and peaceful environment that can help individuals manage their stress levels.
2. Physical activity: Gardening is a form of physical activity that can help individuals stay active and improve overall physical health.
3. Socialization: Gardening can provide opportunities for socialization and community involvement, which can help combat feelings of loneliness and isolation.

4. Sense of accomplishment: Gardening provides a sense of accomplishment and pride in creating and maintaining a beautiful outdoor space.

The Healing Power of Plants

Plants have been used for centuries for their healing properties. In addition to their physical health benefits, plants also have mental health benefits. Exposure to plants has been shown to reduce stress and anxiety and improve overall mood. Plants also have the ability to purify the air, which can improve indoor air quality and overall health.

Gardening as a Form of Therapy

Gardening can be used as a form of therapy to improve mental health. Horticultural therapy is a type of therapy that involves the use of plants and gardening to improve mental health. It has been shown to be effective in reducing symptoms of depression, anxiety, and stress. Horticultural therapy can be done in a group or individual setting, and can involve a range of activities, including planting, harvesting, and caring for plants.

Incorporating Gardening into Mental Health Treatment

Gardening can be incorporated into mental health treatment in a variety of ways, including:

1. Horticultural therapy: As previously mentioned, horticultural therapy can be used as a form of therapy to improve mental health.
2. Community gardening: Community gardening can provide opportunities for socialization and community involvement, which can improve mental health.
3. Home gardening: Simply gardening at home can provide a range of mental health benefits, including stress reduction and a sense of accomplishment.

Conclusion

In conclusion, this chapter has explored the therapeutic benefits of gardening and the healing power of plants. We have discussed how gardening can reduce stress, provide physical activity, and improve socialization. We have also explored how gardening can be used as a form of therapy to improve mental health, including horticultural therapy and community gardening. By incorporating gardening into mental health treatment, individuals can experience the many benefits of gardening and improve their overall well-being. The next chapter will explore the benefits of spending time in nature for addiction recovery.

Chapter 6: Nature and Social Connection

In our modern, technology-driven world, it can be easy to feel disconnected from others. However, spending time in nature can help us reconnect with ourselves and with others. In this chapter, we will explore the connection between nature and social connection and how spending time in nature can improve our relationships and overall well-being.

The Importance of Social Connection

Social connection is a fundamental human need. Humans are social beings, and our relationships with others play a significant role in our overall health and well-being. Social connection has been linked to improved mental health, reduced stress, and improved physical health.

The Connection Between Nature and Social Connection

Spending time in nature can help improve social connection in several ways. These include:

1. Shared experiences: Spending time in nature with others can create shared experiences and strengthen relationships. This can improve feelings of social connection and belonging.

2. Group activities: Many outdoor activities, such as hiking and camping, are best done with others. These group activities can provide opportunities for socialization and create a sense of community.
3. Increased empathy: Exposure to nature has been shown to increase empathy and social awareness. This can lead to more positive social interactions and improved relationships.
4. Mindfulness: Spending time in nature can help individuals become more present and mindful, which can improve communication and social interactions.

Incorporating Nature into Social Activities

Incorporating nature into social activities can provide a range of benefits, including improved social connection and overall well-being. Some ways to incorporate nature into social activities include:

1. Outdoor exercise: Participating in outdoor exercise, such as hiking or biking, with friends can provide both physical and mental health benefits.
2. Nature walks: Taking a leisurely walk in nature with friends can provide an opportunity for socialization and stress reduction.

3. Outdoor picnics: Hosting a picnic in a natural setting can provide a relaxing and enjoyable social experience.
4. Volunteer activities: Participating in outdoor volunteer activities, such as community garden projects or park clean-ups, can provide opportunities for social connection and community involvement.

Conclusion

In conclusion, this chapter has explored the connection between nature and social connection. We have discussed the importance of social connection for overall well-being and how spending time in nature can improve social connection. We have also explored ways to incorporate nature into social activities to enhance socialization and community involvement. By incorporating nature into social activities, individuals can improve their relationships, reduce stress, and improve their overall well-being. The next chapter will explore the benefits of spending time in nature for children's mental health.

Chapter 7: Making Nature a Part of Daily Life

Spending time in nature is beneficial for our mental health and well-being, but it can be challenging to find the time and opportunity to get outside. In this chapter, we will explore ways to make nature a part of our daily lives and reap the benefits of being in nature regularly.

Benefits of Regular Nature Exposure

Regular exposure to nature can provide a range of mental health benefits, including reduced stress, improved mood, and increased creativity. It can also lead to improved physical health, including reduced risk of heart disease and obesity.

Ways to Incorporate Nature into Daily Life

1. Start small: Incorporating nature into your daily routine doesn't have to be a significant undertaking. Start by taking short walks in nature, spending time in a local park, or bringing plants and natural elements into your home.
2. Find natural elements in your environment: Even if you live in an urban area, there are likely natural elements in your environment. Take notice of the

trees, flowers, and green spaces in your neighborhood and take advantage of them.

3. Take advantage of breaks: Instead of scrolling through social media during your breaks, use that time to take a walk outside or sit in a nearby park.

4. Get involved in outdoor activities: Participating in outdoor activities, such as gardening or hiking, can provide a regular dose of nature and improve your overall well-being.

5. Make it a family activity: Spending time in nature with your family can provide a range of mental health benefits for everyone. Plan regular family outings in nature and make it a priority to spend time together in a natural setting.

Conclusion

In conclusion, incorporating nature into our daily lives can provide a range of mental and physical health benefits. By starting small, finding natural elements in our environment, taking advantage of breaks, participating in outdoor activities, and making it a family activity, we can make nature a regular part of our daily routines. By doing so, we can improve our overall well-being and enjoy the healing power of nature. The next chapter will explore the benefits of spending time in nature for older adults.

Conclusion:

The healing power of nature is undeniable. This book has explored the ways in which spending time outdoors can improve mental health, from reducing anxiety and depression to improving cognitive function and creativity. We have discussed the science behind nature, the benefits of nature for specific mental health conditions, the healing power of gardening, and the importance of social connection in nature.

Through these chapters, we have learned that nature has the ability to soothe our minds and bodies, reduce stress, and provide a sense of calm and clarity. Whether it's taking a walk in the park, gardening in your backyard, or hiking in the mountains, there are countless ways to incorporate nature into our daily lives and improve our mental and physical well-being.

As we move forward, it's essential to prioritize spending time in nature, especially as our world becomes increasingly fast-paced and technology-driven. By disconnecting from screens and connecting with nature, we can enhance our mental health and live more fulfilling lives.

In conclusion, the healing power of nature is accessible to all of us. It's up to us to take advantage of it, to step outside and breathe in the fresh air, to listen to the sound of the leaves rustling, and to let ourselves be rejuvenated by the beauty and peace of nature.